# THE PATH TO A
# VIBRANT HEALTH

## A Multi-Dimensional Approach to Health

Joseph Raynauld Raymond

*Doctor of Natural Health*

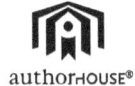

*AuthorHouse™*
*1663 Liberty Drive*
*Bloomington, IN 47403*
*www.authorhouse.com*
*Phone: 1-800-839-8640*

*First published by AuthorHouse    12/29/2011*

*ISBN: 978-1-4678-5712-3 (sc)*
*ISBN: 978-1-4678-5714-7 (e)*

*Library of Congress Control Number: 2011960536*

*Printed in the United States of America*

# CONTENTS

# ACKNOWLEDGEMENTS

Special thanks to my brother Edris for reviewing the text and his encouragement. Thanks to Clayton College of Natural Health Staff for their support and especially to Professor Phyllis Light for her last minute booster that allows me to get my degree. Thanks to my Mom, Marie Ermicile Raymond, for her love and encouragement. Special thanks to my companion in life, Mireille, for her loving support. Thanks to all my brothers, sisters and friends who gave me their full support during my difficult moments in life.

# PREFACE

**The Path to a Vibrant Health** is a book that covers everything that every human being who enjoys a happy and healthy life needs to read. It covers the basic principles of a healthy lifestyle and how to achieve it. In this book, the author teaches us about many different useful resources like fruits, vegetables, exercise and music that are already available to us.

This book offers many great alternatives as to what we need to do in order to maintain our health in good standing. If by any chance you don't have any health issue, this book can still be beneficial to you. You can use it as a preventive guideline.

I am convinced that everyone can learn something from this book. No matter what your health condition is, you can always get some helpful advices from it.

This book is a complete guideline for a better life for those who read, understand and follow **the Path to a Vibrant Health**.

Edris Raymond,
MS. EE; B.Th

# INTRODUCTION

Making good nutritional choices every day is one of the biggest challenges of living a healthy and energetic life. Whole foods are composed of naturally occurring vitamins and minerals, enzymes, fiber, omega-3 essential fatty acids, antioxidants, phytonutrients, and probiotics. These life-giving nutrients give foods their value, color, flavor, and aroma. To stay healthy, we need to provide the body with those essential nutrients. Herbal and nutritional health supplements provide quality ingredients to support our body systems. We must also learn how to cope with the stressors we face in our daily life. In short, we must work to establish the right balance between our mind, body and spirit.

This book, considered as simply educative, is divided into three parts. Part I provides information about nutrition: How to stay healthy by following the basic rules of the nutritional medicine. Part II provides information about herbs functions and properties: How herbs may contribute to our health and well-being. And Part III gives some techniques that may help to manage our daily stressors.

This book is not intended to replace the advices of your Physicians or your healthcare Professionals. The primary goal is to educate and empower you with knowledge that, if applied, will help you in your path to a vibrant health. Your body is yours; it is your own responsibility to take care of it as God intended. "Let food be your medicine and your medicine your food" said the Great Greek Physician Hippocrates, considered as the Father of the Western Medicine.

# PART ONE: NUTRITION.

## I- THE BASELINE OF HEALTH.

Health is defined as a condition in which all functions of the body and mind are normally active. The World Health Organization (WHO) defines health as a state of complete physical, mental, or social well-being and not merely the absence of disease or infirmity.

The body is a whole system and needs to be treated as such. No one organ of the body can be sick without affecting the person as a whole. The practitioners, when working with a client, must assess the totality of the person and must realize that every individual has different needs. We need also to stress that there is no "one size fits all" in our recommendations to clients. The bottom line is that the same supplement used by two different people for the same condition doesn't necessarily produce the same results. In "Biochemical Individuality" by Dr. Roger Williams, 1956, the author showed how in each of us, our organs are of different shapes and sizes, how we have different levels of enzymes, and different needs for protein, vitamins and minerals. And Lucretius said in 50 B.C., "One man's food is another man's poison.

People have different needs but they are general guidelines that everybody can follow in their search of optimum health. Some of them are:

1. Body cleansing and detoxification
2. Hormonal balance
3. Immune system- strengthening
4. Diet

5. Water
6. Exercise
7. Thoughts.

## 1. Body cleansing and detoxification.

A basic program to health must start with a body cleansing and detoxification. Most degenerative diseases come from congestion and stagnation in many parts of the body. This congestion/stagnation state can be cleared from our system through cleansing and detoxification. Many experts agree that health begins in the colon. The intestinal cleansing and detoxification is the "sine qua non" of health.

The colon is the main elimination channel of the body. All the toxic wastes of the digestive process are eliminated through it. The liver considered as the main detoxification organ of the body filters out dangerous drug residues and poisons from the blood and passes them out of the body-through the colon via the bile duct. We can't even begin to cleanse and repair the other systems in the body until we clean out the colon. The toxic wastes must find a clear path to move easily out of the body
The intestinal tract is the source of all nutrient access to our system. It must work properly so that the food we eat can be broken down correctly and our system will benefit of all the nutritional value of the food we eat.

## 2. Hormonal balance.

Hormones are biochemicals produced in special glands and, when present in the bloodstream, give instructions to body cells. For example, Insulin tells the cells to take up glucose from the blood. Thyroxine, from the thyroid gland, speeds up the metabolism of cells, generating energy and burning fat. Estrogen and progesterone, from ovaries, control a sequence of changes that maintain fertility and the menstrual cycle.

The human body has two types of glands: Endocrine glands that have no duct; they secrete their products-hormones- into the circulatory system and Exocrine glands, such as the digestive glands, and sweat glands, which empty their contents through ducts. The endocrine glands, located in various places in the body, secrete hormones. The hormone balance of the body is a complex and interactive symphony of different regulating compounds. The bottom line is to identify and support the glands that must need nutritional support.

The glandular and nervous systems work intimately together to maintain balance among all of the body systems. Together, these systems regulate voluntary and involuntary actions within the body, such as growth, metabolism, digestion, elimination, menstruation and sleep. These systems also serve as the body's means of communication between cells.

They are various lifestyle choices we can make to keep our hormones in balance:
- -Choose organic vegetables and meat wherever possible to reduce pesticide and hormone exposure.
- Exercise regularly
- Reduce the consumption of stimulants such as coffee, tea, chocolate, sugar, and cigarette, if at all.
- Reduce the consumption of animal fats in your diet.
- Make sure you have enough essential fats from seeds or their oils.
- Replace negative thoughts with more positive thoughts.

## 3 Immune system-Strengthening..

The immune system is one of the most remarkable and complex system within the human body. Its purpose is to identify the body's enemies and destroy them. They include defective body cells as well as foreign agents such as bacteria and viruses. The immune system has an army of special cells to deal with invaders. For example, some cells operate in the blood, keeping an eye out for invaders, and whistling up other troops which can destroy specific invaders. The three main types of immune cells found in the blood are: B-cells, T-cells and macrophages, collectively call white cells.

Food choices and diet are considered as major factors in the immune health. However, we must realize that we can't have all the nutrients our immune system needs from food. The American Medical Association (AMA) asserts that everyone should take a multivitamin in order to guard against nutritional deficiencies. Our soil has become so depleted of nutrients that our food does not supply us with nearly as much nutrition as it did 50-100 years ago. It is important to remember that major deficiencies of even one vitamin and mineral can lead to disease. Our immune system can be well supported by providing it with necessary vitamins and minerals, antioxidants, omega-3 fatty acids and probiotics.

## 4. Diet.

Every cell, every organ, and every system in our body benefits from the food we eat. When we eat the highest quality food in the right quantities, we have the ability to achieve our highest potential for health, vitality and freedom from disease. One of the best ways to be healthy is to eat foods that provide exactly the amount of energy we need to keep the body in perfect balance.

We must try to eat organic as much as we can. Raw, organic food is the most natural and beneficial way to nourish our body. An important part of our diet should consist of raw fruits, vegetables, whole grains, nuts and seeds. Processed and refined foods with additives must be avoided as much as we can.

## 5. Water.

Water is the most abundant compound found in our body; it makes up about 60 percent of the body weight of men and about 50 percent of the weight of the women. Water is the primary component of all the bodily fluids. The lymphatic fluid is one of the main areas that house the water in our body. We must drink a sufficient amount of water in order to support the lymphatic system, which in turn facilitate the function of the immune system. Water carries the electrolytes, mineral and salts that help convey electrical currents in the body. The daily need for water consumption varies greatly from person to person. It depends on our activity level, the climate in which we live, and our diet.

## 6. Exercise.

Exercising regularly may help you develop physically and mentally. It is an important factor in our lifestyle change and a key component in our quest for health. By developing an active lifestyle that includes diverse activities, we can

- Lower our blood pressure
- Control our blood sugar and improve our cholesterol levels
- Strengthen our cardiovascular system
- Lose weight or maintain our desire weight
- Facilitate digestion....etc.

Medical research indicates that regular exercise leads to many significant psychological changes such reducing anxiety, tension, and fatigue, relieving depression and increasing vigor and self-esteem. Exercise may also help relieve some negative effects of everyday stress, acting as a buffer against stress-related diseases. In summary, by increasing our physical activities, we can live a better and healthier life.

## 7. Thoughts.

Many health practitioners believe there is a direct connection between our thoughts and the way our immune system functions. Toxic thoughts trigger negative and anxious emotions and thereby produce chemicals that cause the body stress. Intense worry, anxiety, fear, and anger create a strong stress response in the body and can eventually cause the immune system to be less effective in dealing with cancer cells and other types of antigens.

# II- FUNDAMENTALS OF NUTRITION:

Counting calories and comparing the ratios of fat calories to total calories are the essential knowledge for many experts in the nutritional field. In most hospitals, the only concern of the certified nutritionists who prepare hospital "foods" is putting together a correct balance of proteins, fats and carbohydrates. Our source of energy is from food. We need food and its nutrients to live a healthful life. These essential nutrients include the macronutrients- Proteins, fats, and carbohydrates; and the micronutrients-vitamins and minerals.

1. **Proteins** are essential for the growth and repair of all body tissue. Proteins are made of amino acids, some of which our body can produce by itself, and some of which must be included in our diet. Our need for protein is not very large and is easy to fill. The recommended dietary allowance (RDA) of protein according to U.S. government standards is 0.8 gram per kilogram of ideal body weight for adult males and females 19 years and older( 1 kg equals 2.2 pounds).

In Theory, milk is the top-rated protein, in reality it is not. Meat, fish and egg are fine. Some of the best sources, surprisingly, are vegetarian. Spirulina and chlorella are both not only higher in actual percentage of protein (60-80% vs. 20-25% for animal sources) but also in terms of bioviability.

**2. Fats** are the ultimate energy storage system. Our body stores fat for long term energy use. The fats or lipids are found primarily in meats, dairy products, nuts and seeds. Some other vegetable sources of fats include soybeans, olives, peanuts, and avocados. Fats are not only important for energy storage but also required for the transport of other nutrients such as vitamins A, D, E and K the fat-soluble vitamins. Lipids perform many life-supporting functions in each cell of our body. Certain fats are essential for life and health.

- Essential Fatty Acids, or EFA's are among the approximately 50-70 nutrients that have been identified as necessary to sustain human life and good health. Due to the extreme sensitivity of Essential Fatty Acids to light and oxygen, they have been removed from all virtually processed foods so that the foods have a longer shelf life.

- The reason EFA's are so important is that they are the main components of all cellular membranes- inside and out- where they protect against viruses, bacteria, and allergens. They play a key role in the construction and maintenance of nerve cells and the hormonelike substances called prostaglandins and help decrease cholesterol and triglyceride levels in the blood.
- The bottom line is that Essential Fatty Acids are vital to health, although almost 90% of all people are deficient in at least one of them.

**3. Carbohydrates** are the body's short term energy foods. There are many different kinds of carbohydrates but some serve as quick source of energy for the body. Carbohydrates are scientifically classified according to their structure and two basic types of carbohydrates are found in most plant foods. They are free sugars and polysaccharides. Simple carbohydrates, such as sugar and white flour are utilized in the body in a matter of minutes. Complex carbohydrates take much more time to break down and to be utilized by the body. The best foods for carbohydrates are fresh fruits, vegetables, all kinds of beans, peas, lentils, oats, and whole grains. They are high in complex carbohydrate and certain special factors that help release their sugar content gradually. They are also high in fiber, which helps to normalize blood sugar levels as well as assisting the digestive processes.

**4- Vitamins** are co-enzymes whose primary role is to help our body's enzymes do their jobs. The dictionary defines a vitamin as "an organic compound naturally occurring in plant and animal tissue and that is essential in small amounts for the control of metabolic processes". Vitamins are essential in human nutrition. Most vitamins cannot be manufactured in our body. Vitamins are essential for growth, vitality, and health and are helpful in digestion, elimination and resistance to disease. Lack of vitamins can lead to a variety of health problems. Vitamin deficiencies produce well-recognized syndromes (e.g., beriberi- thiamine deficiency- and scurvy- vitamin C deficiency).

Vitamins are usually classified into two categories: water soluble and fat soluble. They are further categorized by letters, groups, and individual chemical names. The water-soluble vitamins include mainly the many B vitamins and vitamin C. Most of the water-soluble vitamins act in the body as coenzymes in combination with an inactive protein to make an active enzyme. And the fat-soluble vitamins are A, D, E, and K with are found in the lipid components of both vegetable and animal sources food (Ref.: table 1: vitamin sources).

**Table 1**: Vitamin Sources

| Vitamins | Sources |
| --- | --- |
| Beta- carotenes | Asparagus, Broccoli, Brussels sprouts, Kale, Lettuce, Mustard greens, Parsley, Seaweed (nori), Spinach, Carrots, Pumpkin, Red cabbage, Sweet potatoes, Yams, Apricots, Cantaloupe, Cherries, Mango, Papaya, Peaches and Watermelon |
| Vitamin B | Brewer's yeast, Beans, Peas, Nuts (Peanut, Brazil nuts, Pecans), Milk, Avocados, Leafy green vegetables,Wheat germ/bran, Rice husks, Blackstrap molasses,Liver and Pork |
| Vitamin C | Citrus fruits (oranges, lemons, limes, tangerines Grapefruits), Rose hips, Acerola cherries, Papayas, Cantaloupe, Strawberries, Red and Green peppers, Broccoli, Brussels sprouts, Tomatoes, Asparagus, Parsley, dark leafy greens and Cabbage |
| Vitamin D | Fish liver oil, Egg yolks, Butter, Liver, Mackerel, Salmon, Sardines and Herring and Sunlight |
| Vitamin E | Cold-pressed vegetable oils (Wheat germ oil, Safflower oil, sunflower oil, Flaxseed oil.), Soybeans, Uncooked green peas, Spinach, Asparagus, Kale, Cucumber, Tomato, Celery |
| Vitamin K | Dark leafy greens, Alfalfa, Kelp, Blackstrap |

molasses, Safflower oil, Liver, Milk, Yogurt, Egg yolks, Fish Liver oils.

**5. Minerals** are essential constituents of all cells; they form the greater portion of the hard parts of the body (bone, teeth, and nails). Our body is made mostly of minerals and water. Our overall health is determined far more by minerals than proteins, fats, carbohydrates or even vitamins. Calcium, for example, is not only used to build strong bones and teeth, but is present in every single cell in the body and is instrumental in the transporting of nutrients in and out of those cells. Although our bodies can manufacture some vitamins, we make no minerals. Our minerals come from the foods we eat. Deficiencies of many vital minerals are common because our body does not make minerals.

There are approximately 17 essential minerals. The seven macro-minerals are calcium (Ca), chloride (Cl), magnesium (Mg), phosphorus (P), potassium (K), sodium (Na), and sulfur (S). And the trace minerals that are know to be essential are chromium (Cr), cobalt (Co), copper (Cu), iodine (I), iron (Fe), manganese (Mn), molybdenum (Mo), selenium (Se), silicon (Si), and zinc(Z). The best approach to get optimal mineral levels is to obtain them from wholesome foods. We need to eat a variety of foods, with a lot of organic, local produce and grains. (Ref. table 2: Essential Mineral Sources)

**Table 2: Essential Mineral Sources.**

| Minerals | Sources |
| --- | --- |
| Calcium (Ca) | Cheese, Yogurt, Cooked broccoli, Sardines With bones), Milk, Almond, Brazil nuts, Tofu, Blackstrap molasses, Parsley, Kelp, Sesame Seeds and Sunflower seeds |
| Chloride (Cl) | Sea salt, Seaweeds (dulce, kelp), Olives, Rye, Lettuce, Tomatoes and Celery |
| Magnesium (Mg) | Dark green vegetables, Nuts (almonds, pecans, Cashews and Brazil nuts), Wheat |

| | |
|---|---|
| | bran/germ, Millet, Brown rice, Tofu, Soy flour, Avocados Dried apricots |
| Phosphorus (P) | Meats, Fish, Chicken, Turkey, Milk, Cheese, Eggs, Seeds, Nuts, Brewer's yeast and Wheat Bran or germ |
| Potassium (K) | Spinach, Parsley, Mustard green, Lettuce, Broccoli, Peas, Lima beans, Tomatoes, Potato skins, Oranges, Bananas, Apples, Avocados, Raisins, Apricots, Wheat germ, Seeds, Nuts, Mushrooms, Fish: (flounder, Salmon, sardines and cod.) |
| Sodium Na) | Celery, Beets, Carrots, Artichoke, Kelp, Beef, Poultry and Seafood |
| Sulfur (S) | Meats, Fish, Poultry, Egg yolks, Milk, Legumes, Onions, Garlic, Cabbage, Brussels sprouts, Kale, Collards, Mustard greens, Chard, Broccoli, Kelp, Lettuce, Turnips, Raspberries |

**6. Trace Minerals** are elements needed by the body in small amounts; many are essential for enzymes functioning. A full complement of the 72-84 trace elements is essential to optimum health. Many of the mineral food level depend on soil content. Table 3 resumes the 10 essential trace minerals and their sources.

**Table 3: Essential Trace Minerals Sources**

| Trace Minerals | Sources |
|---|---|
| Chromium (Cr) | Brewer's yeast, Beef, Liver, Chicken, Oysters, Eggs, Butter, Whole wheat, Rye, Potatoes, Tomatoes, bananas, Spinach, Wheat germ, Black/Green peppers, Onions |
| Cobalt (Co) | Meat, Liver, Kidney, Clams, Oysters, Milk, |

|  | Ocean fish, sea vegetables, Spinach, figs, Lettuce and Cabbage |
|---|---|
| Copper (Cu) | Buckwheat, Whole wheat, Shrimp, Liver, Oysters, Dried peas, Beans, Brazil nuts, Hazelnuts, Pecans, Walnuts and Almonds |
| Iodine (I) | Fish, Shellfish, Sea vegetables, Kelp, Cod, Sea bass, Haddock and Perch |
| Iron (Fe) | Cooked soybeans, Blackstrap molasses, Tofu, Pumpkin seeds, cooked chickpeas, Tempeh, Calf's liver, Prune juice, Raisins, Cashews, Dried figs, Dried Apricots, Potato, Almonds, Cooked Bulgur, Sesame seeds, Sunflower seeds, Prunes, Watermelon |
| Manganese (Mn) | Romaine lettuce, Kale, Mustard green, Spinach, Alfalfa, Black teas, Coffee beans, Seeds, Nuts and Egg yolks |
| Molybdenum (Mo) | Oats, Buckwheat, Wheat germ, Lima beans, Green beans, Lentils, Potatoes, Spinach, Cauliflower, Peas, Soybeans, Brewer's Yeast and Liver |
| Selenium (Se) | Brewer's yeast, Wheat germ, Whole grains, Brazil nuts, Molasses, Barley, Oats, Whole Wheat, Brown rice, Salmon, Snapper, Halibut, Scallops, Lobsters, Shrimp, clams, Crab, Oysters, Garlic, Onions, Broccoli, Mushrooms, Tomatoes, Radishes |
| Silicon (Si) | Wheat, Oats, and Rice hulls, Sugar beet, Sugar cane pulp, alfalfa, Horsetail, comfrey, Nettles, Lettuce, Cucumber, Avocados, Strawberries, Onions, Dandelion, Dark Greens, Kelp, Pectin (citrus fruits) |

| Zinc (Zn) | Oysters, Red meats (beef, lamb and pork), Liver, Herring, Egg yolks, Poultry, milk, Whole wheat, Rye, Oats, Pecans, Brazil nuts, Pumpkin seeds, Ginger root, Mustard, Chili powder, Black pepper, Peas, Carrots, Beets, Cabbage |
|---|---|

**7. Phytochemicals** are the hot "new" discoveries in nutritional science. They are biologically active compounds in food; they are not classified as nutrients, in that our lives do not depend on them as they do for vitamins. However, they do play a vital role in the body's biochemistry in ways that affect our health as significantly as vitamins and minerals. As they are not stored in the body it is best to eat foods rich in phytochemicals on a regular basis. More than one hundred phytochemicals have been identified; some of them are:

- **Allium compounds**. Members of the allium family include: garlic, onions, leeks, chives and shallots.
- **Bioflavonoid**s. They include: rutin (lots in buckwheat) and hesperidin found in citrus fruits. The best food sources are rosehips, buckwheat leaves, citrus fruits, berries, broccoli, cherries, grapes, papaya, cantaloupe, plums, tea, red wine, cucumber, and tomatoes.
- **Capsaicin**. It is abundant in hot peppers.
- **Chlorophyll**. This is the substance that makes green plants green. It is found in wheat, grass, seaweeds, and green vegetables.
- **Coumarins and chlorogenic Acid**. These substances are found in a variety of fruits and vegetables including tomatoes, green peppers, pineapple, strawberries, and carrots.
- **Ellagic Acid**. It is found in strawberries, grapes and raspberries.
- **Isothiocyanates (ITCs) and Indoles**. These are plentiful in what are known as the cruciferous vegetables, which include broccoli, brussels sprouts, cabbage, cauliflowers, cress, horseradish, kale, mustard, radishes, and turnips.
- **Phytoestrogens**. Foods rich in phytoestrogens include: soybeans, wheat, licorice, alfalfa, fennel and celery.
- **Sulforaphane**. It is found in broccoli, cauliflower, Brussels sprouts, turnips and kale.

**8. Enzymes** are considered the keys of life. We always repeat "we are what we eat". Well, not quite- we are what we can digest and absorb. The food we eat cannot nourish us unless it is first prepared for absorption in the body. This is done by enzymes, chemical compounds which digest it and break down large food particles into smaller units. Protein is broken down into amino acids; complex carbohydrates into simple sugar; and fat into fatty acid and glycerol.

The three main families of digestive enzymes are amylases, which digest carbohydrate; proteases, which digest protein; and lipases, which digest fat. As an aid to digestion, many nutritional supplements contain these enzymes.

**9. Antioxidants** are chemicals capable of disarming free radicals. Some are known essential nutrients like vitamin A and beta-carotene, and vitamin C and E. Others, like bioflavonoids, anthocyanidins, pycnogenol, and over a hundred other recently identified protectors found in common foods, are not.

Free radicals are made in all combustion processes including smoking, the burning of gasoline to create exhaust fumes, radiation, frying or barbecuing food and normal body processes.

Antioxidants are found in nature, including substances in berries, grapes, tomatoes, mustard and broccoli and in herbs such as turmeric and ginkgo biloba. Beta-carotene is found in red/orange/yellow vegetables and fruits. Vitamin C is also abundant in vegetables and fruits eaten raw, but heat rapidly destroys it. Vitamin E is found in "seed" foods, including nuts, seeds and their oils, vegetables like peas, broad beans, corn, and whole grains. Antioxidants keep energy flowing in a manner that prevents damage to the cells and tissue. Table 4 resumes some Antioxidant Nutrients and Herbs.

**Table 4: Some Antioxidant Nutrients and Herbs**

| Nutrients | Herbs |
|---|---|
| Vitamin C (Ascorbates, Ascorbate Esthers) | Aloe vera |
| Vitamin E (Tocopherols, Tocotrienols) | Bilberry |
| Lutein | Garlic |
| Selenium | Green tea |
| Sulfur | Ginkgo |

Carotenoids

Lipoid acid

Coenzyme Q10 (Coq10)

Flavonoids (hesperidin, quercetin, rutin)

Carnosine

Hawthorn

Milk thistle

Mangosteen

Goji Berries

Acai berries

Pomegranate

Noni

Indian Gooseberry

Turmeric

**10. Fiber** is indigestible carbohydrate. This is a natural constituent of a healthy diet high in fruits, vegetables, lentils, beans and whole grains. By consuming such high fiber diet, we are at less risk of colon cancer, diabetes, and diverticular diseases and are unlikely to suffer from constipation. An ideal intake of fiber is not less than 35 grams a day. It is probably best to get fiber from a mixture of sources such as oats, lentils, beans, seeds, fruits and raw or lightly cooked vegetables. According to the U.S. Department of Agriculture's 2010 Dietary Guidelines for Americans, most Americans don't get enough fiber. The guideline states that dietary fiber is a nutrient of public health concern in American diets and suggests choosing foods that provide more fiber.

# III- YOUR OPTIMUM DIET

Diet is the essential key to all successful healing. Without a proper balance diet, the effectiveness of herbal treatment is very limited. For a simple diet, the intake of foods can be divided into three categories:

## Primary foods:
-   Whole grains (Wheat, Oats, Barley, Maize, Brown rice, Rye, Amaranth, Quinoa…etc) may constitute about 20%- 30% of the diet.
-   Protein, such as tofu, tempeh and beans, including animal protein, 20%- 30% of the diet. Vegetable sources of protein must be consumed in larger amount to equal a corresponding amount of animal protein. Beans must be consumed in small amount because of their high carbohydrate content.

Whole grains, because of their high fiber content, take more time for their absorption by our systems and do not trigger our insulin. In traditional societies, such as those in China, India, Japan and Central America, whole grains and beans constitute a therapeutic diet that accompany any kind of treatment.

## Secondary foods:
Fresh vegetables (mostly lightly cooked)-may constitute about 30% -40% of the diet. The secondary foods are fresh, local, seasonal vegetables, which provide important vitamins and mineral nutrients. When we need to eliminate toxins from our body and have eaten too much meat and processed foods, vegetables such as fresh salads may be used to start the healing process.

## Tertiary foods:
-   Fruits, dairy and eggs -5%-10% of the diet; lipids such as olive oil, canola oil, and sesame oil- 2%.

We must give ourselves the best possible intake of nutrients to allow the body to be as healthy as possible and to work as well as it can. Everybody has different needs in term of nutrition. No one diet is perfect for everyone.

**A daily diet tip** may consist of the followings:

1- One tablespoon of ground seeds or one tablespoon of cold-pressed seed oil
2- Three servings of fresh fruit such as: bananas, pears, apples, melon, berries or citrus fruit.
3- Two servings of lentils, beans, quinoa, tofu, or "seed" vegetables.
4- Four servings of whole grains such as brown rice, oats, rye, millet, whole wheat, or corn
5- Four servings of dark green, leafy and root vegetables such as carrots, spinach, sweet potatoes, broccoli, cauliflower, asparagus, green beans, peas or peppers.
6- A minimum of 64 ounces of pure, ph optimized water.
7- Eat whole, organic, raw food whenever you can
8- Supplement your diet with a high-strength multivitamin and mineral preparation.
9- Avoid refined, processed foods of all kinds, hydrogenated fat, and excess animal fat.
10- Minimize your intake of alcohol, coffee and tea.

We are going to talk about two types of diet that many experts in nutrition considered as healthy ones. They are: Macrobiotic diet and Mediterranean diet.

# IV- MACROBIOTIC AND MEDITERRANEAN DIETS.

The **Macrobiotic movement** in U.S. was initiated by Mr.Michio Kushi., the founder of the Kushi Institute in Becket, Massachusetts. Mr. Kushi's mentor in Japan thought that food was the key to health and that health was the key to peace. He believed that humanity would regain its physical and mental balance and become more peaceful by returning to a traditional diet of whole, natural foods. The term "Macrobiotic" is Greek for "great life" or "long life" Hippocrates used the term to describe people who are healthy and lived long. Other classical writers used the term to describe a lifestyle, including a simple, balance diet that promoted health and longevity.

In general, Macrobiotics emphasizes locally grown whole cereal grains, legumes, vegetables, seaweed, fruits and fermented foods combined into meals according to the principle of balance known as yin and yang.

The **Mediterranean diet** is rich in cereals, fruits, vegetables, nuts, whole grains, fish and olive oil. People who live in the Mediterranean have a much lower risk of cardiovascular disease. While their diet contains lots of fruits, vegetables and fish, their lower incidence of heart disease has been correlated with their high intake of olive oil, a source of monounsaturated fat. Another reason to use olive oil is that it contains myriad of minor components that have major health benefits. These include phytosterols, chlorophyll, magnesium, vitamin E and carotenes. Vitamin E and magnesium in particular are vital for good cardiovascular health.

For instance, findings published in the European Journal of clinical Nutrition report that a diet rich in olive oil, and fruits and vegetables was associated with a significant reduction in the incidence of hypertension. One thing to remember is that you must buy extra virgin (unrefined) olive oil to obtain these health advantages.

# V- WHY DO WE NEED SUPPLEMENTS?

People, even if they are eating a normal diet, may be diagnosed deficient in certain nutrients. These are some of the reasons:

1-The foods we eat today are not as rich in nutrients as the foods that our grand-parents ate 50-100 years ago.
   a) Often fruits are picked before they are ripe, so they can last longer during transportation. They are ripened artificially before they are put on the shelves. Crops picked before they are fully developed may not have the time to reach their peak level of nutrients.
   b) When we process foods, they are ripped of some of their essential nutrients.
   c) Soils are not rich in minerals as they once used to be. Soils are depleted of some nutrients because of the use of chemicals and pesticides in the agriculture. Since crops largely gain their nutrients from the soil, low nutrient levels in the soil means low nutrient levels in the food.

2- People with certain conditions don't absorb optimally nutrients from the foods they eat. For examples, people with gut inflammation, food intolerances, and poor digestive function have problems of absorption

3- Other factor to consider is nutritional stress. We are exposed to far more environmental and pollution stresses than we can tolerate. Our bodies were never designed to handle:
   - High levels of refined and processed foods
   - High levels of radiation
   - A totally fiberless white flour diet
   - Constant exposure to disruptive electromagnetic fields
   - High-stress jobs and living situations.

The bottom line is that supplements can play a major role in the maintenance of good health. We need food supplements to reduce the risk of cancer, heart disease, degenerative diseases of all kinds. We must remember that food supplements are not food replacements; they must be taken together with a Wholistic healthy diet and a lifestyle change for best results.

He causes the grass to grow for the cattle, and vegetation for the service of man. That he may bring forth food from the earth (Psalm 104:14-The New King James Version Bible).

# PART TWO: HERBAL SUPPLEMENTATION

## I- THE FUNCTIONS OF HERBS

Medicinal plants have been used for centuries to keep us healthy. The art of using herbs as medicine has stood the test of time and continues today with the school of Natural Health. Nowadays, according to statistics, Million of Americans are seeking advices from alternative health Practitioners as medical costs are skyrocketing and the side effects of chemical drugs are alarming.

Herbs are our most natural and potent healers. They gently and very effectively can help by nourishing and strengthening our body. Herbs work on the cause of the problem rather than just the symptoms. In this way, once a problem is corrected, it should not recur. Herbs have three general functions in the body and are compounded according to the state of the individual. We can use herbs to cleanse and detoxify the body by using eliminative herbs that work as laxatives, diuretics, diaphoretics and blood purifiers. We can use herbs for maintenance of our body by using herbs that counteract the physical symptoms and allowing the body to heal itself. And we can use herbs for building our systems by using herbs that tone the organs.

Our bodies are comfortable with herbs, recognize them, and utilize them efficiently. While allopathic medicine provides only relief for symptoms, herbs act on the causes of the diseases and heal for ever. It looks like they act at the cellular level.

# II- HERBAL PREPARATION

Herbal preparations are available in many different forms: teas, tinctures, fluid extracts, and bulk herbs, powdered herbs in capsules and tablets, and solid extracts. Herbs can also be used as poultices, compresses, salves and oils.

a) **Teas:** Practitioners of herbal medicine have often used a form of medicinal tea called *decoction*. A decoction is made by combining bulk herbs in water and boiling them together. The mixture is then strained and the liquid consumed. Decoctions are very concentrated medicinal teas. And we have *infusion* made by pouring boiling water over the herb and letting it steep. Tea bags are the most common form of infusion used in America.

b) **Tinctures:** A tincture is made by letting an herb soak in a solvent (usually alcohol or water) for several hours, days, even weeks depending on the herb. Tinctures are most commonly made with alcohol. Sometimes, glycerin has been used to make alcohol-free" tinctures but the preparation is not as good as the tinctures with alcohol. Tinctures are typically a 1:5 or 1:10 concentration. This means that one part of the herbal material is prepared with five or ten parts (by weight) of the liquid.

c) **Fluid extracts:** Fluid extracts are more concentrated than tinctures. They are often made with either alcohol or water, but sometimes other solvents may be used in an extraction. Fluid extracts are typically a 1:1 concentration.

d) **Solid extracts:** A solid extract is the most concentrated form of an herbal product. It results when all of the solvent is evaporated off, leaving a solid residue. These residues are usually available in powdered form. Solid extracts are typically 2:1 to 8:1 concentrations.

e) **Herbal powders:** Herbal powders, usually available in capsules or tablets, have minimal processing.

f) **Standardized extracts:** Standardized extracts have become popular among health care practitioners because they allow for more consistency in dosing. Standardization means guaranteed levels of a certain constituent or group of constituents in the final product. This quality is usually expressed as a percentage of the total weight of the extract.

g) **Poultices and compresses.** A poultice is a wad of chopped, fresh plant material that is applied directly to a wound or infection on the skin and held in place by a wet dressing that is covered by a bandage. Poultices work primarily at the application site, typically preventing infection and speeding the healing of the wounds. Compresses are clean clothes that have been dipped in an herbal solution- an infusion, decoction, tincture or vinegar. You might hold a poultice in place with a compress. In this case, it doubles like a bandage. Or you might apply it directly to the skin (fomentation).

h)  **Salves**. Making salves involves mixing medicinal herbs with water, beeswax, animal fat, vegetable fat and other ingredients to create spreadable lotions. First, you cover the pulverized herb with water. Then boil or simmer for 15 to 30 minutes. Let it cool. Add some oil, and then gently heat the oily mixture until the water is evaporated, perhaps 15 to 30 minutes. Finally, add beeswax and /or a fat to give your salve the proper consistency. Cool before using.

i)  **Oils.** One of the methods to prepare oils is by macerating and pounding the fresh or dried herbs in a mortar or pestle. Olive oil or sesame oil is then added (one pint oil to two ounces of herb) and the mixture is allowed to stand in a warm place for three days. Then the oil is strained and bottled. Oils are frequently made from spices, mints and other aromatic herbs.

# III- HERBAL PROPERTIES

Each herb has a combination of specific effects on particular systems of the body, and also some very general effects. It is possible to confront the entire scope of the disease by carefully matching the herbal properties with the symptoms being treated. Every herb has hundreds of biochemical constituents that lend themselves to descriptions according to their physiological effects, or properties. These properties are widely accepted by Natural Health Practitioners who used herbs in their Practice. Some herbs will end up in more than one category. Some of the properties are:

1. **Alteratives (blood purifiers).** Some alteratives include: alfalfa, aloe vera, red clover, dandelion root, burdock root, cascara sagrada, echinacea, goldenseal, uva ursi and Oregon grape. These agents gradually and favorably alter the condition of the body. They are used in treating toxicity of the blood; helped the body to assimilate nutrients and eliminate waste products of metabolism.
2. **Analgesics.** Analgesics include: chamomile, cramp bark, cloves, catnip, don quai, lobelia, kava kava, skullcap, valerian and wild yam. These herbs are taken to relieve pain without causing loss of consciousness.
3. **Antacids.** Dandelion, fennel, aloe vera, slippery elm, irish moss, and kelp function as antacids. They help to neutralize excess acids in the stomach and intestines.
4. **Antiasthmatics.** Antiasthmatics include: mullein, lobelia, yerba santa, colts foot, wild yam, comfrey, elecampane and wild cherry bark. These agents help relieve the symptoms of asthma.
5. **Antibiotics.** Antibiotic herbs include: Echinacea, goldenseal, myrrh, chaparral, buchu, juniper berries, garlic and thyme. The substances in these herbs helped inhibit the growth of, or destroy, bacteria, viruses, or amoebas.
6. **Antipyretics.** Antipyretics include: alfalfa,basil, boneset, gotu kola, skullcap, chickweed and the seaweeds. They are cooling herbs that used to reduce or prevent fevers. Cooling may refer to neutralizing harmful acids (excess heat) as well as reducing body temperature.
7. **Antiseptics.** Antiseptics include: calendula, chaparral,

goldenseal, myrrh, and the oils of thyme, garlic, pine, juniper berries, and sage. They are substances that can be applied to the skin to prevent the growth of bacteria.

8. **Antispasmodics.** Antispasmodics include: chamomile, black cohosh, don quai, skullcap, motherwort, mullein, passion flower, valerian, kava kava, raspberry leaves and peppermint. These substances can be applied either internally or externally to relax the muscles.

9. **Aphrodisiacs.** Aphrodisiacs include: damania, ginseng, kava kava, false unicorn, angelica, astragalus and burdock. They are substances used to increase sexual power and excitement.

10. **Astringents.** Astringents include: horse chestnut, witch hazel, white oak bark, bayberry bark, calendula, juniper berries, pomegranate, pau d'arco, squaw vine and stoneroot. Tannins are the primary component of herbal medicines commonly labeled "astringent". Tannin-containing herbs are useful in treating inflammation of the skin and mucous membrane. Externally, tannins are also useful to speed wound healing. Internally, tannins add tone to the gastrointestinal (GI) tract, helping stop diarrhea and soothing irritated tissue.

11. **Carminatives.** Carminatives include: chamomile, peppermint, fennel, dill, cumin, caraway, anise, ginger, thyme and calamus. These herbs soothe and tone the digestive system. They are high in volatile oils and are used in cases of GI upset, irritation and cramping. They helped relieve excess gas and bloating.

12. **Cholagogues.** Cholagogues include: dandelion root, artichoke, goldenseal root, chelidonium, milk thistle, turmeric, aloe vera, barberry, licorice and Oregon grape root. These herbs helped to stimulate the production of bile and the proper flow of bile. By improving bile production and flow, these herbs also reduce the risk of gallstone formation. They are also associated with improving fat digestion and promoting healthy liver function.

13. **Demulcents.** Demulcents include: aloe vera, fenugreek seeds, slippery elm, marshmallow root, mullein flowers, plantain leaves, burdock, licorice, chickweed, and flax. These herbs are high in mucilage. They are noted for their ability to soothe or protect irritated mucous membranes inside the body. A

demulcent herb is commonly referred to as an *emollient* when applied topically to the skin.

14. **Diaphoretics.** Diaphoretics include: chamomile, ginger, cayenne, elecampane, elder flowers, yarrow flowers, lemon balm, catnip, boneset and hyssop. They are herbs that induce perspiration.

15. **Diuretics.** Diuretics include: dandelion, fennel, feverfew, foxglove, horsetail, parsley, agromony, uva ursi, cleaversand buchu. They are herbs that increase the secretion and flow of urine.

16. **Emetics.** Emetics include: black mustard seed, ipecac, lobelia, elecampane, boneset, blessed thistle, foxglove, elder, wintergreen, and pansy. They are substances that induce vomiting and cause the stomach to empty.

17. **Emmenagogues.** Black cohosh, myrrh, rue, angelica, pennyroyal, juniper berries, and wild yam are emmenagogues. They are herbs that promote menstruation, usually, causing it to occur earlier, and sometimes with increase flow.

18. **Expectorants.** Eucalyptus, anise, foxglove, licorice, lobelia, mullein, elecampane, yerba santa, colsfoot, and wild cherry bark are expectorants. These herbs assist in expelling mucus from the lungs and throat.

19. **Galactologues.** Anise seed, blessed thistle, fennel, cumin, and vervain are galactologues. These herbs help to increase the secretion of milk.

20. **Hemostatics.** Hemostatics include: bayberry, cayenne, mullein, goldenseal, horsetail, white oak bark, yellow dock, witch hazel , yarrow and sheperd's purse. These substances are used to stop hemorrhaging.

21. **Laxatives.** Cascara bark, rhubarb root, aloe vera, psyllium seed, flax seed, chia seed, senna, castor oil, slippery elm, and Oregon grape are laxatives. They are substances that promote bowel movements.

22. **Nervines.** Nervines include: wild cherry, chamomile, passion flower, skullcap, lobelia, valerian, lady's slipper, nettle, wood betony and fu ling. These substances assist in calming the nervous tension and nourishing the nervous system.

23. **Sedatives.** Sedatives include: chamomile, passion flower, marigold, valerian, skullcap, catnip, wood betony, kava kava,

mugwort and yarrow. These herbs are used to strongly quiet the nervous system.

24. **Sialogogues.** Echinacea, black pepper, cayenne, ginger, licorice and yerba santa are sialogogues. They are substances that stimulate the flow of saliva and thus aid in the digestion of starches.

25. **Stimulants.** Stimulants include: anise, cayenne, black pepper, cinnamon, Echinacea, ginseng, sarsaparilla, dandelion, angelica, ginger, garlic and astragalus. They are herbs that increase the energy of the body, drive the circulation, break up obstruction and warm the body.

26. **Tonics.** Tonics include: boneset, wild cherry, damania, dandelion, devil's claw, blessed thistle, yarrow, yellow dock, sarsaparilla and ginseng. They promote the functions of the systems of the body.

27. **Vulneraries.** Vulneraries include: aloe vera, cayenne, comfrey, fenugreek, garlic, calendula, rosemary, thyme, marshmallow and slippery elm. These herbs encourage the healing of wounds by promoting cell growth and repair.

# IV- TRENDS IN THE USE OF HERBS

A survey conducted by Eisenberg et al in 1990 affirms that an estimate of one-third of the U.S. adult population was using some form of alternative medicine. When similar survey was conducted in 1997, they found that estimated expenditures for alternative medicines services increased by 45.2 percent and were estimated at $ 21.2 billions. Of this large amount, over one-half was paid out of pocket. Compared with 1990, the largest increase in use for any therapy was herbal medicine, which now ranked second. The survey suggests that an estimated fifteen millions adults in the United States are using herbal or nutritional supplements with prescription medications.

Another event that contributed to the growth of herbal supplement market was the passage of the Dietary Supplement and Health Education Act (DSHEA) at the end of 1994. DSHEA was a blessing for both the supplement industry and consumers. Suddenly, labels were able to make claims that told you what an herb really does in the body. They describe the way an herb or herbal constituent influences or supports body structure or function. An FDA ruling on February 7, 2000 actually expands the scope of structure-function claims that can be made for herbal and nutritional supplements.

These days, it looks like the herbal medicine has fallen into a new category named "Complementary and Alternative Medicine" (CAM). Information about herbs and CAM has exploded in the past years. Consumers are avid of information. Many journals, even the mainstream medical Journals published articles on herbal medicines and CAM. Over two-third of all U.S medical schools offered courses on CAM, which helped doctors answer patient's questions. As mainstream medicine becomes more interested in herbal medicine, one of the payoffs will be increased opportunities for clinical studies. There is a bright future for the growth of herbal medicine in the United States.

And He showed me a pure river of water of life, clear as crystal, proceeding from the throne of God and of the Lamb. In the middle of its street and on either side of the river was the tree of life, which bore twelve fruits, each tree yielding the fruit every month. The leaves of the tree were for the healing of the nations (Revelation 22: 1, 2- The New King James Version Bible).

# PART THREE: STRESS MANAGEMENT.

## 1- SOURCES OF STRESS.

Stress can be defined as any change to which you must adapt. Stress and tension are present in your daily life. Stress management and relaxation can be effective only if you make them a daily part of your lifestyle. It is how you respond to the stressful events of your daily life that determines the impact of stress on your life. You experience stress from four basic sources:

1. You must adjust to the demands of your environment. You must adapt to the weather, pollens, noise, traffic and air pollution

2. You must also deal with social stressors such as job interviews, work presentations, interpersonal conflicts, financial problems, and the loss of loved ones.

3. The third source of stress is physiological. The rapid growth of adolescence, the changes menopause causes in woman, illnesses, injuries, and aging, all tall tax your body. Your physiological reaction to environmental and social threats and changes also can result in stressful symptoms such as headaches, stomach upset, muscle tension, anxiety and depression.

4. The fourth source of stress is your thoughts. Your brain interprets complex changes in your environment and your body and determines when to turn on the "stress response".

Researchers have been looking at the relationship between stress and diseases for over a hundred years. They have observed that people suffering from stress- related disorders tend to show hyperactivity in a particular preferred system" or " stress-prone system", such as gastrointestinal system, cardiovascular, or skeletomuscular system. For instance, chronic stress can result in muscle tension and fatigue for some people. For others, it can contribute to stress hypertension (high blood pressure, migraine headaches, ulcers, or chronic diarrhea). Almost every system in the body can be damaged by stress.

## II. SOME TECHNIQUES TO COPE WITH STRESS.

There is a tendency to think of stressful events or stressors only as negative (such as the injury or the death of a loved one) but stressors are often positive. For instance, getting a new job or promotion at work brings with it the stress of change of situations and new responsibilities. You can increase your ability to deal with negative stress or distress by integrating in your daily life positive activities such as solving challenging problems, practicing regular exercise workouts and relaxation techniques, staying in touch with enjoyable social contacts and engaging in optimistic and rational thinking. The following practices are very helpful in managing your daily stressors:

1. **Breathing.** You can use breathing to reduce or to eliminate the symptoms of stress and to release tension and relax. Breathing is the fundamental necessity of life. With each breath of air, you obtain oxygen and release the waste product: carbon dioxide. Poor breathing habits diminish the flow of these gases to and from your body making it harder for you to cope with stressful situations. Conversely, breath awareness and good breathing habit may enhance your psychological and physical well-being.

When you breathe, typically you use one of the two patterns: chest or thoracic breathing, or abdominal or diaphragmatic breathing. Chest or thoracic breathing is a common malady of modern life that is often linked with lifestyle, stress, anxiety, or other forms of emotional distress. It is shallow and often irregular and rapid; whereas, abdominal or diaphragmatic breathing is the natural and normal breathing. It is deeper and slower than shallow chest breathing, as well as more rhythmic and relaxing. The respiratory system is able to do its job of producing energy from oxygen and removing waste products.

Breathing exercises have been found to be effective in reducing generalized anxiety disorders, panic attacks, depression, irritability, muscle tension, headaches and fatigue.

2. **Exercises**. Exercise is a simple and effective way to manage stress. Any form of exercise may counteract your body's natural stress response.

Exercise releases endorphins into your bloodstream creating a sense of well-being. It decreases muscle tension caused by emotional stress and produce a relaxation response in your mind as well as in your body. There are three categories of exercise: aerobic/cardiovascular, stretching/flexibility, and toning/strengthening.

-Aerobic exercises involve sustained use of the large muscles in the body, especially in your legs and arms. The goals of aerobic exercise are to strengthen your cardiovascular system and to increase your overall stamina. Popular aerobic exercises include: running, jogging, brisk walking, swimming, bicycling and dancing.

-Stretching and toning exercises are used to increase muscle strength and flexibility and to maintain healthy joints. Stretching exercises are slow, sustained and relaxing. To be effective, a stretch needs to be held steady for at least thirty seconds. Stretching decreases muscle tension, improves circulation, and helps prevent injury when used during the warm-up and cool-down periods before and after aerobic exercise.

Toning exercises utilize higher repetitions and lower weights to target muscles that need firming. Some examples of toning exercises are crunches for stomach muscles, squats for thigh muscles, heel raises for calf muscles, and push-ups for arms and chest muscles.

3. **Laughing**. Laughter reduces emotional and physical tension by producing an internal massage. Laughing stimulates your circulatory, respiratory, vascular and nervous systems. Laughter takes your attention off yourself and your situation. It provides you with the distance necessary to gain perspective on a situation that you may be taking too seriously.

4. **Massage.** Massage is one of the oldest healing arts. Persians and Egyptians applied forms of massage for many ailments; and Hippocrates wrote many papers recommending the use of rubbing and friction for joint and circulatory problems. Stress relief is the key to achieving a healthier lifestlyle. Massage can significantly lower heart rate, cortisol and insulin levels- all of which help reduce daily stress. Massage boosts the body's immune system, which can become compromised from extended periods of stress.

**5. Meditation.** Meditation is the intentional practice of focusing your attention on one thing at a time. The meditator repeats, either loud or silently, a syllable, word, or a group of words. This is known as mantra meditation. You can use anything as an object of meditation. With regular meditation, a person feels more focused and calm in her life, more capable of making new choices in the moment, and less prone to engage in struggle and reactive responses. Meditation has been used successfully in the treatment and prevention of high blood pressure, heart disease, migraine headaches, and autoimmune diseases such as arthritis and diabetes. It has been proved helpful in curtailing obsessive thinking, anxiety, depression, and hostility.

**6. Music.** Listening to music is one of the most common forms of relaxation. It is important, therefore, that when you want to listen to music for the purpose of relaxation, you select music you find peaceful and soothing.

# CONCLUSION

Since the beginning of time, people have relied on plants as foods and medicines. Herbs are more effective in addressing the underlying causes of imbalance in the body than the prescription drugs with all the side effects that everybody knows. Foods, like medicines, are best used in their natural matrix, so whole foods are more nutritious and assimillable. We need to approach the problems wholistically when working with clients. We must remember the interconnection between the body, mind and spirit. The natural medicine doesn't consider the individual as a set of symptoms but as a whole person looking for correcting the imbalance in his systems-whether it is physical, emotional or spiritual.

Understanding our inner healing power is the first step toward correcting the imbalance in our systems. If we provide our body with all the necessary nutrients, it has the ability to heal itself. We must be conscious of the necessity to listen to our body and to take back our health. Nobody can know our body better than us. We believe, one day, the American people will be able to choose the health care system that correspond to their needs; they will have the freedom to choose between the traditional medicine and the natural medicine for their care or the integration of both. I believe in the near future, the health insurance companies will give the opportunity to its subscribers to receive the care from the system of their choice.

I would like to take this opportunity to share my own experiences in using plants in my daily life. I was using the antacid drugs (Maalox, Gelusil, Tums, Pepsid, Nexium…etc) for more than 20 years. I remember that I was sitting in the consultation room at my primary doctor's office when I asked her this question "When will I stop taking the Nexium?" I was really tired taking these pills. She just smiled because she had no answer. Since, I started to search on the internet for any alternative. I found an herb that I used by following the instructions. The first day I start taking the herb, I put away the Nexium. In my curiosity, I found other herbs that I used to control my cholesterol that the doctor found too high. I believed that for all diseases God has created some plants. That is the reason why I am now a natural health consultant with the option to use plants for my foods and medicines. Plants work wonder if we use patience and perseverance.

# APPENDIX A:
## Foods for Specific Body Parts.

**Adrenals:**
- **Herbs:** Astragalus, Evening primrose oil, Ginger, Ginseng, Juniper, Licorice root, Lobelia, Milk Thistle, and Parsley
- **Vegetables:** Asparagus, All leafy greens, Legumes, Lima beans, Mushrooms, Okra, Olive oil, Onions, Red pepper, and Sprouts
- **Fruits:** Blueberries, Coconut, Figs, Gooseberries, Grapefruit, Lemons, Oranges, Prunes and Strawberries
- **Nuts/Grains/Seeds:** Almonds, Brown rice, Flaxseed, Millet, Molasses, Wheat bran/germ, and wild rice

**Bladder:**
- **Herbs:** Buchu leaves, Cornsilk, Elder flowers, Horsetail, Juniper berries, Nettle, Oatstraw, Parsley and Uva usi
- **Vegetables:** Broccoli, Cauliflower, Cabbage, Green beans, Lettuce, Parsley, Potato skin, Red/Green peppers and Spinach
- **Fruits:** Acerola cherries, Apples, Blueberries, Cantaloupe, Cranberries, Grapefruit, Lemons, Strawberries, and Watermelon
- **Nuts/Grains/Seeds:** Almonds, Brown rice, Flaxseed, Molasses, Oats, Soybeans, Sunflower seeds, Wheat bran/germ

**Bones:**
- **Herbs:** Alfalfa, Boneset, Dandelion root, Garlic, Horsetail, Nettles, Pokeroot, and Rose hips
- **Vegetables:** All leafy greens, Asparagus, Broccoli, Brussels Sprouts, Cabbage, Cauliflower, Kale, Lettuce, Lima beans, Mushrooms, Onions, Sea vegetables and Watercress.
- **Fruits:** Apples, Acerola cherries, Bananas, Blueberries, Cantaloupe, Figs, Kiwi, Gooseberries, Grapefruit, Lemons, Oranges, Peaches, Prunes, Red grapes, and Strawberries
- **Nuts/Grains/Seeds:** Almonds, Filberts, Flaxseed, Molasses, Oats, Sesame seeds, Soybean, Sunflower seeds, and Wheat germ.

## Brain/Nerves:
- **Herbs:** Alfalfa, Cayenne, Ginkgo biloba, Ginseng, Gotu kola, Kelp, Lobelia, Parsley, Skullcap, St.John's wort, and Valerian root
- **Vegetables:** All leafy greens, Avocados, Beans, Broccoli, Cabbage, Cauliflower, Chickpeas, Corn, Lentils, Lettuce, Potatoes, Red/Green peppers, Reishi mushrooms, Soybeans, Spinach, and Tomatoes
- **Fruits:** Blackberries, Blueberries, Cantaloupe, Coconut, Grapefruit, Orange, Pineapples, Prunes, and Strawberries
- **Nuts/Grains/Seeds:** Almonds, Barley, Flaxseed, Millet, Molasses, Oats, Pecans, Rice bran, Rye, Sesame seeds, and Wild rice.

## Bronchi:
- **Herbs:** Astragalus, Black radish, Cayenne, Eucalyptus, Fenugreek, Garlic, Ginger, Lobelia, Mullein, Myrrh, Parsley, and Peppermint.
- **Vegetables:** All leafy greens, Asparagus, Avocados, Broccoli, Cabbage, Cauliflower, Green beans, Lentils, Mushrooms, Onions, Potatoes, Sprouts, and Tomatoes.
- **Fruits:** Apples, Blackberries, Black cherries, Cranberries, Gooseberries, Grapefruit, Peaches, Prunes, and Strawberries
- **Nuts/Grains/Seeds:** Almonds, Barley, Millet, Molasses, Oats, Peanut with skin, Pecan, Rice bran, Sesame seeds, Sunflower seeds, and Wild rice

## Eyes:
- **Herbs:** Alfalfa, Bilberries, Chamomile, Eder flowers, Eyebright, Garlic, Ginkgo biloba, Golden seal, Horsetail, Nettle, and yarrow
- **Vegetables:** All dark leafy greens, Beans, Broccoli, Carrots, Cauliflower, Chickpeas, Lettuce, Onions, Pumpkin, Red/Green peppers, Spinach, Squash, Sweet potatoes, and Tomatoes
- **Fruits:** Apricots, Blueberries, Cantaloupe, Cranberries, Dates, Figs, Peaches, Prunes, and Strawberries
- **Nuts/Grains/Seeds:** Almonds, Flaxseed, Oats, Pumpkin seeds, Rye, Sunflower seeds, Wheat bran/germ.

## Female Reproductive Organs:
- **Herbs:** Black/Blue cohosh, Damania, Don quai, False unicorn, Horsetail, Kelp, Licorice root, Nettle, Primrose oil, Rasberry, Sarsaparilla, Saw palmetto, Uva ursi, and White oak bark
- **Vegetables:** Asparagus, Cabbage, Celery, Cucumbers, Ginger root, Mushrooms, Red peppers, Sea vegetables, Spinach, and Watercress
- **Fruits:** Acerola berries, Apples, Cantaloupe, Figs, Grapefruits, Oranges, and Strawberries
- **Nuts /Grains/Seeds**: Alfalfa, Flaxseed, Molasses, Oats, Pumpkin seeds, Sunflower seeds, Wheat germ.

## Gall Bladder:
- **Herbs:** Barberry, Burdock, Dandelion, Fenugreek, Gentian root, Golden seal, Kelp, Mandrake, White oak bark
- **Vegetables:** Broccoli, Cauliflower, Carrots, Lettuce, Radish, Red/Green peppers, Spinach, Sweet potatoes, and Tomatoes
- **Fruits:** Apples, Black berries, Lemons, Pears, and Pineapples
- **Nuts/Grains/Seeds**: Flaxseed, Oats, Olive oil, Sunflower seeds, Wheat, Wheat germ.

## Gums/Teeth:
- **Herbs:** Garlic, Ginger, Golden seal, Lobelia, Myrrh, Oatstraw, Sage tea, Tea tree oil, and Valerian root.
- **Vegetables**: Bok choy, Broccoli, Cabbage, Cauliflower, Carrots, Kale, Lettuce, Mushrooms, Red/Green peppers, Spinach, and Wheatgrass.
- **Fruits:** Apricots, Apples, Bananas, Cranberries, Figs, Goosberries, papaya and Prunes.
- **Nuts/Grains/Seeds**: Almonds, Brown rice, Flaxseed, Millet, Sesame seeds, and Wheat bran/germ.

## Hair/Scalp:
- **Herbs**: Alfalfa, Cayenne, Dandelion, Ginkgo biloba, Horsetail, Kelp, Nettle, Oatstraw, Primrose oil, and Sage.
- **Vegetables:** Asparagus, Beans, Lentils, Broccoli, Carrots, Cauliflower, Lettuce, Watercress, Red/Green peppers, Sea vegetables, Spinach, and Sweet potatoes.

- **Fruits:** Apples, Bananas, Cranberries, Dates, Grapefruits, Gooseberries, Oranges and Prunes.
- **Nuts/Grains/Seeds**: Almonds, Brown rice, Flaxseed, Millet, Mushrooms, Oats, Rye flour, Sesame seeds, Sunflower seeds, Wheat, Wheat germ.

## Heart:

- **Herbs:** Garlic, Black cohosh, Cayenne pepper, Ginkgo biloba, Gotu kola, Hawthorn berries, Horsetail, Linden flowers, Shitake and Yarrow.
- **Vegetables**: Artichoke, Avocados, Asparagus, Broccoli, Cabbage, Carrots, Cauliflower, Eggplant, Kale, Kelp, Onions, Spinach, Sweet potatoes, Yam, Tomatoes, Watercress, and Yellow squash.
- **Fruits:** Apricots, Apples, Bananas, Black berries, Blueberries, Dates, Figs, Kiwi, Cantaloupe, Papaya, Peaches, Red grapes.
- **Nuts/Grains/Seeds**: Almonds, Barley, Brown rice, Buckwheat, Flaxseed, Millet, Molasses, Oats, Oat bran, Olive oil, Psyllium seeds, Rice bran, Sesame seeds, Soybean, Sunflower seeds, and Wheat germ.

## Intestines:

- **Herbs:** Alfalfa, Aloe vera, Chamomile, Fennel, Fenugreek, Garlic, Golden seal, Licorice root, Pau d'arco and Psyllium seds.
- **Vegetables:** Beans, Beets, Cabbage, Carrots, Celery, Chard, Cucumber, Dandelion, Lentils, Lettuce, Okra, Olives, Onions, Parsley, Spinach, Tomatoes, and Turnips.
- **Fruits**: Cantaloupe, Figs, Gooseberries, Grapefruit, Papaya, Peaches, Pineapple, Prunes, and Strawberries.
- **Nuts/Grains/Seeds**: Almonds, Brown rice, Flaxseed, Millet, Oat bran, Rice bran, Soybean and Wheat germ.

## Joints:

- **Herbs:** Alfalfa, Cayenne pepper, Garlic, Horsetail, Kelp, Nettle, Primrose oil, and Yucca.
- **Vegetables:** Beans, Beets, Cabbage, Carrots, Celery, Collards, Cucumber, Dandelion, Lentils, Lettuce, Olives, Onions, Spinach, Sea vegetables, and Turnips.
- **Fruits:** Bananas, Blueberries, Coconut, Figs, Gooseberries, Grapefruit, Lemons, Peaches, Prunes, Strawberries, Watermelon.

- **Nuts/Grains/Seeds**: Almonds. Flaxseed, Lentils, Oats, Pumpkin seeds, Rice bran, Soybeans, Wheat, Wheat bran/germ.

## Kidneys:
- **Herbs:** Burdock, Cornsilk, Dandelion root, Ginkgo biloba, Juniper berries, parsley leaves and root, Slippery elm, Shiitake tea, Uva ursi and White oak bark.
- **Vegetables:** Beans, Beets, Cabbage, Carrots, Celery, Cucumber, Dandelion, Kale, Lentils, Lettuce, Olives, Onions, Parsley , Shiitake mushroom, Spinach and Turnips.
- **Fruits:** Bananas, Blueberries, Coconut, Cranberries, Figs, Gooseberries, Grapefruit, Lemons, Peaches, Prunes, Strawberries and Watermelon.
- **Nuts/Grains/Seeds**: Alfalfa, Almonds, Brown rice, Oats, Pumpkin seeds, Rice bran, Soybeans, Wheat, and Wheat bran/germ.

## Liver:
- **Herbs:** Astragalus, Barberry, Black radish, Burdock root, Cascara sagrada, Dandelion, Echinacea, Fenugreek, Garlic, Milk thistle, Suma, Red clover, Schizandra, Thyme and Yellow dock.
- **Vegetables:** All leafy greens, Artichoke leaf, Asparagus, Beets, Brussels sprouts, Cabbage, Carrots, Celery, Cucumbers, Dandelion, Endive, Okra, Onions, Reishi mushrooms, Radishes, Spinach, Turnips and Watercress.
- **Fruits:** Apples, Black berries, Black cherries, Figs, Gooseberries, Grapefruit, Grapes, Oranges, Papaya, Peaches, Prunes, and Strawberries.
- **Nuts/Grains/Seeds**: Almonds, Barley, Brown rice, Corn germ, Lentils, Oats, Oat bran, Peanuts, Soybeans, Sunflower seeds, and Wheat bran/ germ.

## Lungs:
- **Herbs:** Coltsfoot, Eucalyptus, Fenugreek, Garlic, Licorice root, Lung wort, Marshmallow, Mullein, Myrrh, Nettle, Reishi, Rosehips, Sage and Slippery elm.
- **Vegetables:** All leafy greens, Asparagus, Beets, Cabbage, Carrots, Celery, Cucumber, Dandelion, Endive, Horseradish, Kale, Okra, Onions, Potato skin, Spinach, String beans, Tomatoes, Turnips and Watercress.

- **Fruits:** Apricots, Bananas, Black berries, Black cherries, Blueberries, Cantaloupe, Coconut, Cranberries, Figs, Grapefruit, Gooseberries, Oranges, Papaya, Peaches, Prunes **and Strawberries.**
- **Nuts/Grains/Seeds:** Almonds, Barley, Brown rice, Corn germ, Flaxseed, Lentils, Millet, Molasses, Oats, Peanuts, Sesame seeds, Soybeans, Sunflower seeds and Wheat germ.

## Lymphatics:
- **Herbs:** Black radish, Burdock root, dandelion, Echinacea, Garlic, Milk thistle, Poke root, Red clover, and Schizandra.
- **Vegetables:** Asparagus, Beets, Cabbage, Carrots, Celery, Cucumber, Dandelion, Horseradish, Okra, Onions, String beans and Turnips.
- **Fruits:** Bananas, Figs, Blueberries, Peaches, Prunes, Strawberries and Watermelon.
- **Nuts/Grains/Seeds:** Almonds, Brown rice, Flaxseed, Oats, Pumpkin seeds, Sunflower seeds, Wheat and Wheat germ.

## Male Reproductive Organs:
- **Herbs:** Cayenne, Chickweed, Chlorophyll, Ginkgo biloba, Ginseng, Kelp, Raspberry, Saw palmetto, Nettle and Pygeum.
- **Vegetables:** Asparagus, Beets, Cabbage, Cauliflower, Green/Red peppers, Lettuce, Okra, Onions, Parsnips, Radishes, Spinach and Tomatoes.
- **Fruits:** Apricots, Figs, cranberries, Dates, Gooseberries, Prunes and Strawberries.
- **Nuts/Grains/Seeds:** Almonds, Barley, Brow rice, Millet, Oats, Pumpkin seeds, Wheat, and Wheat germ/bran.

## Mammary Glands/Breasts:
- **Herbs:** Black walnut, Don quai, Ginkgo biloba, Gotu kola, Horsetail, Kelp, Marshmallow, and Saw palmetto.
- **Vegetables:** Asparagus, Beets, Broccoli, Cabbage, Celery, Lettuce, Okra, Onions, Parsnips, Radishes, Spinach, and Tomatoes.
- **Fruits:** Apricots, Figs, Cranberries, Dates, Gooseberries, Prunes and Strawberries.
- **Nuts/Grains/Seeds:** Alfalfa, Almonds, Barley, Brown rice, Oats, Millet, Soybeans, Sunflower seeds, Wheat and Wheat bran/germ.

## Muscles:
- **Herbs:** Horsetail, Juniper berries, Korean ginseng, Mexican yam. Nettle, Rosemary, Sarsaparilla, St. John's wort and Valerian root.
- **Vegetables:** Alfalfa, All leafy greens, Asparagus, Beans, Cabbage, Lettuce, Lentils, Onions, Parsnips, Radishes, Reishi mushrooms, Spinach and Tomatoes.
- **Fruits:** Apricots, Black figs, Cranberries, Prunes and Strawberries.
- **Nuts/Grains/Seeds**: Almonds, Barley, Brown rice, Flaxseed, Millet, Oats, Sesame seeds, Soybeans, Sunflower seeds and Wheat bran/germ.

## Nails:
- **Herbs:** Alfalfa, Eucalyptus, Horsetail, Kelp, Mullein, Nettle and Peppermint.
- **Vegetables:** Asparagus, Beets, Bok choy, Cabbage, Lettuce, Onions, Parsnips, Radishes, Sea vegetables, Spinach, Soybeans and Tomatoes.
- **Fruits:** Cherries, Coconut, Cranberries, Dates, Figs, Gooseberries, Plums, Prunes and Strawberries.
- **Nuts/Grains/Seeds:** Almonds, Barley, Brown rice, Flaxseed, Oats, Sesame seeds, Sunflower seeds and Wheat bran/germ.

## Pancreas:
- **Herbs:** Alfalfa, Dandelion, Ginseng, Goldenrood, Goldenseal, Horsetail, Huckleberries, Juniper berries, Nettle and Red clover.
- **Vegetables:** Asparagus, Beets, Bok choy, Cabbage, Celery root, Green beans, Kale, Okra, Onions, Parsnips, Peas, Radishes, Spinach, Sea vegetables, Tomatoes, Turnips and Watercress.
- **Fruits:** Apricots, Bananas, Cranberries, Dates, Gooseberries, Papaya, Pineapple, Prunes and Strawberries.
- **Nuts/Grains/Seeds:** Almonds, Barley, Flaxseed oil, Oats, Pumpkin seeds, Sunflower seeds, Wheat bran/germ.

## Prostate:
- **Herbs:** Alfalfa, Buchu, Bee pollen, Burdock root, Goldenseal, Juniper berries, Nettle **and Saw palmetto.**
- **Vegetables**: Asparagus, Beets, cabbage, Lettuce, Onions, Parsnips, Radishes, Spinach, and Tomatoes.

- **Fruits:** Bananas, Coconut, Cranberries, Dates, Figs, Gooseberries, Kiwi, Prunes and Strawberries.
- **Nuts/Grains/Seeds:** Barley, Flaxseed, Oats, Pumpkin seeds, Sunflower seeds, and Wheat bran/germ.

## Skin:
- **Herbs**: Alfalfa, Aloe vera Burdock root, Dandelion, Garlic, Horsetail, kelp, Nettle, Raspberry leaves and Yellow dock.
- **Vegetables:** All leafy greens, Avocados, Beets, Broccoli, Carrots, Celery, Cucumber, Kale, Kidney beans, Lentils, Pumpkin, Sea vegetables, Spinach, Squash and Sweet potatoes.
- **Fruits:** Apples, Apricots, Bananas, Blueberries, Cantaloupe, Cherries, Figs, Lemons, Papaya, Peaches, Prunes, Red grapes and Watermelon.
- **Nuts/Grains/Seeds**: Brown rice, Millet, Oat bran, Pumpkin seeds, Rice bran, Soybeans and Wheat germ.

## Thyroid:
- **Herbs**: Alfalfa, Burdock root, Dandelion, Dulse, Garlic, Ginseng, Goldenseal, Horsetail, Kelp and Sage.
- **Vegetables**: Asparagus, Beets, Brussels sprouts, Cabbage, Carrots, Cauliflower, Celery, Dandelion, Okra, Onions, Parsley, Potato skin, Sea vegetables, Turnips and Yellow corn.
- **Fruits:** Apricots, Black berries, Black cherries, Blueberries, Coconut, Cranberries, Dates, Figs, Gooseberries, Grapefruit, Oranges, Peaches and prunes.
- **Nuts/Grains/Seeds:** Almonds, Barley, Molasses, Oatmeal, Soybeans, Sunflower seeds, Walnuts, Wheat germ and Yeast.

## Uterus:
- **Herbs:** Alfalfa, Bayberry, Black and Blue cohosh, Don quai, False unicorn, Goldenseal, Horsetail, Kelp, Licorice root, Primrose oil, Sage and Sqaw vine.
- **Vegetables:** All leafy greens, Beans, Beets, Brussels Sprouts, Cabbage, Carrots, Cauliflower, Lettuce, Onions, Parsnips, Potato skin, Sea vegetables, Soybeans, Spinach, Tomatoes and Watercress.
- **Fruits:** Apricots, Black berries, Black cherries, Figs, Gooseberries, Prunes Red raspberries and Strawberries.

- **Nuts/Grains/Seeds**: barley, Flaxseed, Oats, Pumpkin seeds, Sunflower seeds, Wheat bran/germ.

## Veins /Arteries:
- **Herbs:** Alfalfa, Buckwheat, Butcher's broom, Cayenne, Hawthorn berries, Kelp, Nettle, White oak bark and Yarrow.
- **Vegetables**: All leafy greens, Asparagus, Beets, Cabbage, Carrots, Celery, Dandelion, Endive, Lettuce, Mushrooms, Okra, Onions, Parsnips, Spinach, Turnips and Watercress.
- **Fruits:** Apricots, Black berries, Black cherries, Blueberries, Cranberries, Dates, Figs, Gooseberries, Grapefruit, Oranges, Peaches, and Prunes.
- **Nuts/Grains/Seeds:** Almonds, Barley, Buckwheat, Chestnuts, Flaxseed, Molasses, Pumpkin seeds, Soybeans, Sunflower seeds, Walnuts and Wheat germ.

# APPENDIX B:
## Commonly Recommended Herbal Medicines.

| Common name | Latin name | Properties |
|---|---|---|
| Alfalfa | Medicago sativa | Nutritive tonic, Antipyretic, Diuretic, Antianemic, Antihemorrhagic. |
| Aloe vera | Aloe vera | Cholagogic, Laxative, Antidiabetic,Cathartic, Stomachic, Vulnerary. |
| Artichoke | Cynara Scolymus | Hepatic, Cholagogic, Diuretic, Antirheumatic, Digestive, Anticholesterol. |
| Astragalus | Astragalus membranaceus | Stimulant, Tonic, Diuretic |
| Bilberry | Vaccinium myrtillus | Astringent, Refrigerant, Diuretic. |
| Black cohosh | Cimicifuga racemosa | Antispasmodic, Expectorant, Emmenagogue, Diaphoretic, Alterative, Nervine. |
| Boneset | Eupatorium perfoliatum | Febrifuge, Diaphoretic, Expectorant, Laxative. |
| Burdock | Articum lapa | Nutritive, Diuretic, Alterative, Diaphoretic. |
| Cascara sagrada | Rhamnus purshiana | Bitter Tonic, Laxative, Nervine, Emetic. |
| Cayenne | Capsicum anuum | Astringent, Carminative, Stimulant, Antispasmodic. |

| Chamomile | Matricaria chamomilla | Stomachic, Nervine, Anodyne, Carminative, Antispasmodic, Diaphoretic, Emmenagogue. |
|---|---|---|
| Chasteberry | Vitex agnus castus | Emmenagogue, Tonic |
| Cinnamom | cinnamomum zeylanicum | Stimulant, Stringent, Demulcent, Carminative. |
| Cranberry | Vaccinium macrocarpon | Lithotriptic |
| Dandelion | Taraxacum officinale | Cholagogue, Diuretic, Tonic, Stomachic, Aperient, Alterative. |
| Echinacea | Echinacea angustifolia | Echinacea Purpurea Antibiotic, Sialogogue, Stimulant. |
| False Unicorn | Chamaelirium luteum | Uterin Tonic, Diuretic, Anthelmintic, Vermifuge. |
| Fennel | Foenicolum vulgare | |
| | Foenicolum officinale | Carminative, Antacid, Galactogogue. |
| Fenugreek | Trigonella foenum- | |
| | Graecum | Astringent, Demulcent, Tonic, Emollient, Expectorant. |
| Feverfew | Tanacetum parthenium | |
| | Chrysanthemum parthenium | Stomachic, Diuretic, Antispasmodic. |
| Garlic | Allium sativum | Alterative, Diaphoretic, Stimulant, Expectorant, Antibiotic, Carminative. Vulneraries, Antispasmodic. |
| Ginger | Zingiber officinale | Stimulant, Diaphoretic, Antispasmodic, Digestive, Anti-inflammatory. |
| Ginkgo | Ginkgo biloba | Expectorant, Antitussive, Antiasthmatic, Sedative. |

| Hawthorn | Crataecus oxycantha | Diuretic, Astringent Nerve Tonic. |
|---|---|---|
| Horse Chestnut | Aesculus hippocastanum | Febrifuge, Narcotic, Tonic |
| Kava Kava | Piper methysticum | Stimulant, Diuretic, Antispasmodic, Analgesic, Anticonvulsant, Anesthetic. |
| Licorice | Glycyrrhiza glabra | Cholagogue, Sialagogue |
| Milk Thistle | Silybum marianum | Bitter Tonic, Antdepressant, Hepatoprotective, Demulcent. |
| Mullein | Verbascum Thapsus | Expectorant, Antitussive, Antispasmodic, Demulcent. |
| Noni | Morinda citrifolia | Antibacterial, Alterative, Antiparasitic, Stomachic, Emmenagogue, Anticancer, Antihypertensive, Analgesic. |
| Passionflower | Passiflora incarnate | Antispasmodic, Anodyne, Hypotensive, Hypnotic. |
| Red Clover | Trifolium pretense | Alterative, Expectorant, Antispasmodic, Antitumor. |
| St. John's Wort | Hypericum perforatum | Astringent, Antidepressant, Sedative, Antiinflammatory |
| Saw Palmetto | Serenoa repens | Diuretic, Expectorant, Sedative, Aphrodisiac. |
| Siberian Ginseng | Eleutherococcus Senticocus | Antirheumatic, Tonic, Antispasmodic. |
| Turmeric | Curcuma longa | Cholagogue, Alterative, Emmenagogue, Analgesic, Astringent, Antiseptic. |

| Valerian | Valerian officinalis | Hypnotic, Sedative, Nervine, Carminative, Antispasmodic, Stimulant, Anodyne. |
|----------|----------------------|------------------------------------------------------------------------------|

**ALFALFA**
Medicago sativa

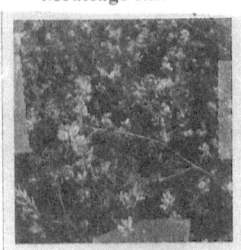

**ALOE VERA**
Aloe vera

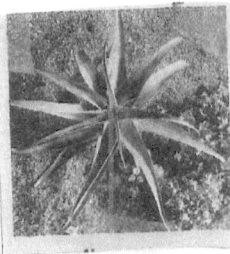

**ARTICHOKE**
Cynara scolymus

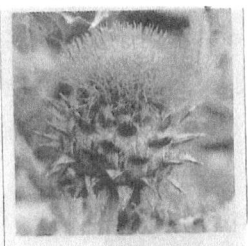

**ASTRAGALUS**
Astragalus membranaceus

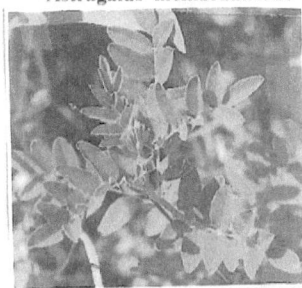

**BIBERRY**
Vaccinium myrtillus

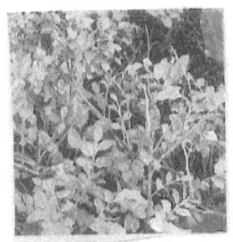

**BLACK COHOSH**
Cimifuga racemosa

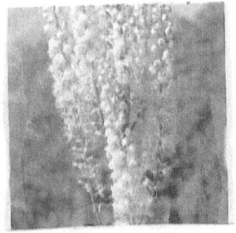

**BONESET**
Eupatorium perfoliatum

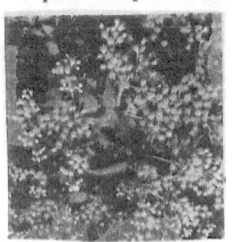

**BURDOCK**
Articum lapa

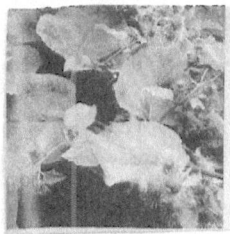

**CASCARA SAGRADA**
Rhamnus purshiana

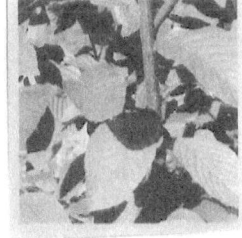

**CAYENNE**
Capsicum annuum

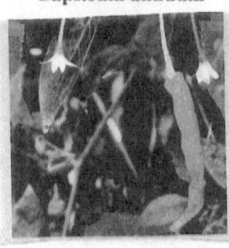

**CHAMOMILE**
Matricaria chamomilla

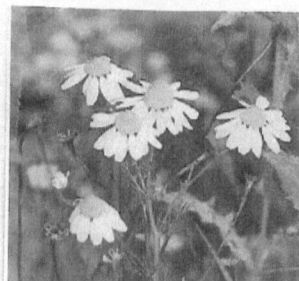

**CHASTEBERRY**
Vitex agnus-castus

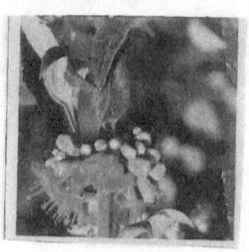

**CINNAMON**
Cinnamomum zeylanicum

**CRANBERRY**
Vaccinium macrocarpon

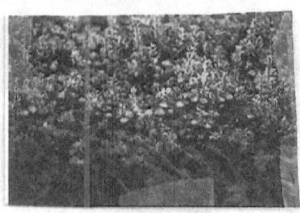

**DANDELION**
Taraxacum officinale

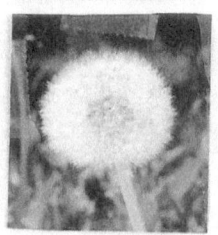

**ECHNACEA**
Echinacea purpurea

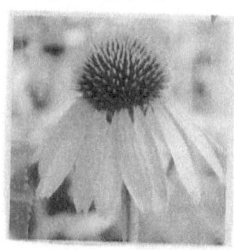

**FALSE UNICORN**
Chamaelirium luteum

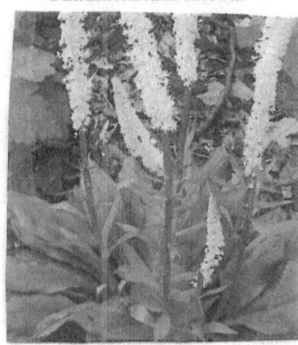

**FENNEL**
Foeniculum vulgare

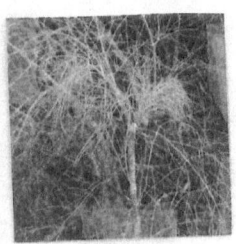

**FENUGREEK**
Trigonella foenum-graecum

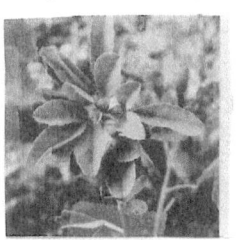

**FEVERFEW**
Tanacetum parthenium

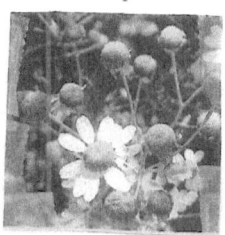

**GARLIC**
Allium sativum

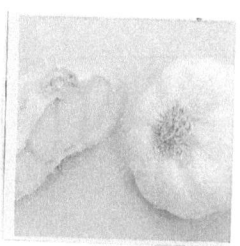

**GINGER**
Zingiber officinale

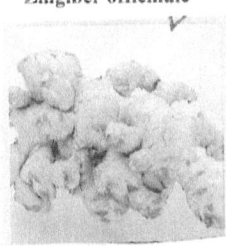

**GINKGO**
Ginkgo biloba

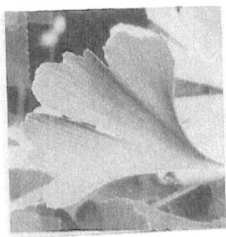

**HAWTHORN**
Crataecus oxycantha

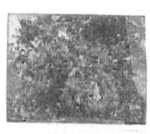

**HORSE CHESTNUT**
Aesculus hippocastanum

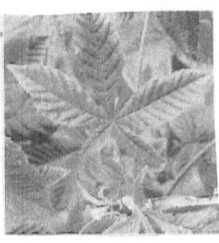

**KAVA KAVA**
Piper methysticum

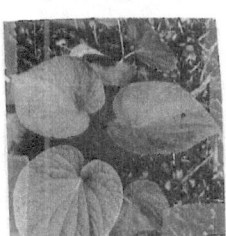

**LICORICE**
Glycyrrhiza glabra

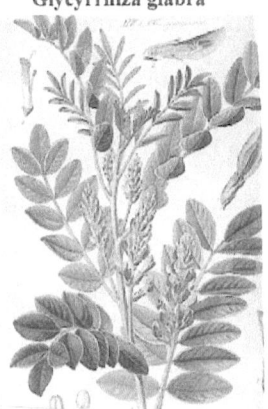

**MILK THISTLE**
Silybum marianum

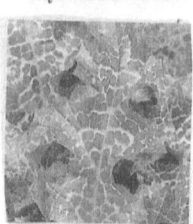

**MULLEIN**
Verbascum thapsus

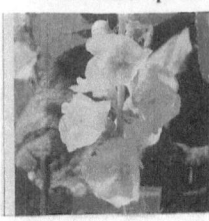

**NONI**
Morinda citrifolia

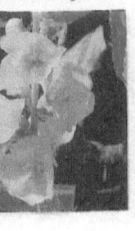

**PASSION FLOWER**
Passiflora incarnata

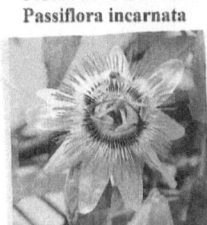

**RED CLOVER**
Trifolium pratense

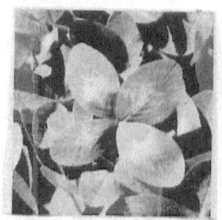

**ST.JOHN'S WORT**
Hypericum perforatum

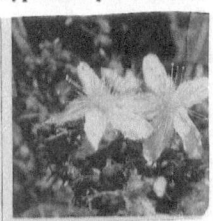

**SAW PALMETTO**
Serenoa repens

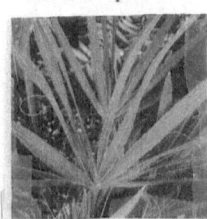

**SIBERIAN GINSENG**
Eleutherococcus senticocus

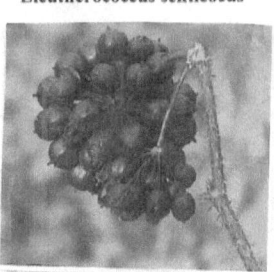

**TURMERIC**
Curcuma longa

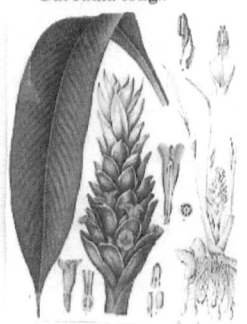

**VALERIAN**
**Valerian officinalis**

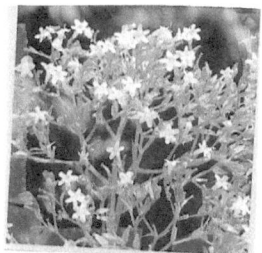

# BIBLIOGRAPHY

-Balch, J. F. & Stengler, M. (2004). *Prescription for natural cures: A self-care guide for treating diseases and health problems with natural remedies including diet and nutrition, herbal medicine, nutrition supplements, bodywork, and more.* Hoboken, NJ: John Wesley & Sons.

- Balch, P. A. & Balch, J. F. (1992). *Prescription for dietary wellness using foods to heal.* Garden City Park, NY: Avery Publishing Group.

- Barron, J. (2022). *Lessons from the miracle doctors: A step-by-step guide to optimum health and relief from catastrophic illness.* Laguna Beach, CA: Basic Health Publications.

- Brown, D. J. (2000). *Herbal prescription for health & healing.* Twin Lakes, WI: Lotus Press.

- Davis, M., Eshelman, E. R. & McKay, M. (2008). *The relaxation & stress reduction workbook.* Oakland, CA: New Harbinger Publications.

-Duke, J. A.(1997). *The green pharmacy: New discoveries in herbal remedies for common diseases and conditions from the world's foremost authority on healing herbs.* Emmaus, PA: Rodale Press.

- Foster, S. & Tyler, V. E. (1999). *Tyler's honest herbal: A sensible guide to the use of herbs and related remedies.* Binghamton, NY: Haworth Herbal Press.

- Gladstar, R. (1993). *Herbal healing for women: Simple home remedies for women of all ages.* New York, NY: A fireside Book.

- Griggs, B. (1997). *Green pharmacy: The history and evolution of western herbal medicine.* Rochester, VT: Healing Arts Press.

-Haas, E. N. & Levin, B. (2006). *Staying healthy with nutrition: A complete guide to diet and nutritional medicine.* Berkley, CA: Celestial Arts.

-Holford, P. (1999). *The optimum nutrition bible*. Freedom, CA: The Crossing Press.

- Kloss, J. (1949). *Back to Eden*. Loma Linda, CA: Back to Eden Books.

-Mabey, R., McIntyre, M., Pamela, M., Duff, G. & Stevens, J. (1988). *The new age herbalist*. New York: A Fireside Book.

-Mowrey, D. B. (1986). *The scientific validation of herbal medicine*. Illinois: Cormorant Books.

-Patton, D. (2004). *Mountain medicine: The herbal remedies of Tommie Bass*. Birmingham, AL: Natural Reader Press.

-Tierra, M. (1998). *The way of herbs*. New York, NY: Pocket Books.

- Theiss, P. & Theiss, B. (1989). *The family herbal*. Rochester, VT: Healing Arts Press.

- Weiner, M. A. & Weiner, J. A. (1994). *Herbs that heals: Prescription for herbal healing*. Mill Valley, CA: Quantum Books.